WORDS *of* HOPE *and* HEALING

THE
GRIEF *of*
INFERTILITY

Alan D. Wolfelt, Ph.D.

Companion
PRESS

An imprint of the Center for Loss and Life Transition | Fort Collins, Colorado

Companion Press is an imprint of the Center for Loss and Life Transition, 3735 Broken Bow Road, Fort Collins, Colorado 80526.

25   24   25   22   21   20   6   5   4   3   2   1

ISBN: 978-1-61722-291-7

CONTENTS

WELCOME

"There is a unique pain that comes from preparing a place in your heart for a child that never comes."

— David Platt

As you know so deeply, infertility is not only an ongoing physical struggle. For many, it's also a years-long emotional, social, and spiritual journey that can take you through countless highs and lows, hopes and disappointments, interspersed with long, painful valleys of uncertainty.

We as a culture aren't very helpful when it comes to supporting people experiencing the grief of infertility. I'm sorry for that. In this book, I hope to help open a door that is too often closed, if only just a little. If you have struggled with infertility, you deserve better. You deserve your experiences to be heard. You deserve your thoughts and feelings to be affirmed. You deserve to be comforted and supported. And you deserve to hear more about the actions you yourself can take to integrate your normal and natural grief into your ongoing life.

Yes, integrating your grief is possible, whether you are still trying to have a baby, have had a baby but are still mourning pregnancy loss or infertility experiences, or are no longer pursuing pregnancy. I have been a grief counselor and educator for more than forty years, and I have companioned a number of families knocked down by infertility. They have taught me that not only can you survive what may at times seem unsurvivable, you can go on to create a life of meaning and joy. I have been privileged to learn from them, and in this book I will share their hard-won wisdom with you.

Thank you for entrusting me to companion you on your journey of heartbreak and hope.

YOU ARE NOT ALONE

"After years of buying baby gifts for others, one in eight people wonder if it will ever be their turn."
— Author unknown

Infertility is at once a common experience and the most intimate and singular of losses.

Today, one in eight women suffers infertility, which as you know is defined as a condition of the reproductive system that inhibits or prevents conception after at least a year of unprotected sex (six months if the woman is 35 or older). If you consider couples, the infertility rate climbs even higher, to one in six. And in women over 35, infertility affects one in three.

In short, infertility affects hundreds of millions of people the world over, and where there is infertility, there is infertility grief.

It's also important for us to remember that infertility affects both women and men. About a third of infertility experiences are due to biological fertility problems in men, while another third are due to biological fertility problems in women. The remainder are caused by a combination of male and female issues as well as those with no clear cause, which can be particularly frustrating. Regardless of its origin, women grieve infertility, and men grieve infertility too.

In addition, many people struggle with primary infertility, meaning they have never had a child, while others find themselves stymied by secondary infertility, meaning they have had a child but find themselves unable to have another.

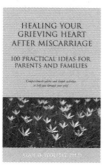
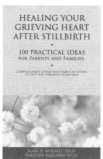

FOR MISCARRIAGE AND STILLBIRTH

If you have suffered a stillbirth or miscarriage(s), I believe you will find the content in this small resource helpful, but it is likely that you also have natural mourning needs and concerns that go beyond its scope. I have written more extensive books on these unique types of loss, and I encourage you be supported by them as well.

Find them at **www.centerforloss.com**

What's more, for some, infertility lasts for a period of difficult years later followed by the birth of a child. For others—including but not limited to those with congenital reproductive challenges (such as physical abnormalities or obstacles associated with transgender reproduction), permanent or premature infertility caused by illness or trauma (such as endometriosis or issues caused by cancer treatments), or running out of time (such as deciding to pursue pregnancy later in life or premature menopause)— infertility is a forever loss.

What's essential to understand in all of this is that women and men in all of these types of infertility circumstances often grieve deeply and deserve support and empathy. No matter your unique infertility story, your grief is real and valid. I see you, and I welcome you to this conversation.

If you have longed for and tried to have a biological child of your own but have, for whatever reason, been unable to have a baby, you are experiencing infertility grief.

You are not alone. The millions of others affected by infertility are all around you. Finding ways to be open about and support one another in your shared grief will help everyone.

AN INVISIBLE GRIEF

*"The English language lacks the words to mourn an absence.
For the loss of a parent, grandparent, spouse, child, or friend,
we have all manner of words and phrases. We are conditioned
to say something, even if it is only 'I'm sorry for your loss.'
But for an absence, for someone who was never there at all,
we are wordless to capture that particular emptiness. For those who
deeply want children and are denied them, those missing babies
hover like silent ephemeral shadows over their lives. Who can
describe the feel of a tiny hand that is never held?"*

— Laura Bush

Let's talk for a moment about what grief is.

Grief is everything you think and feel inside of yourself after
you lose something you are attached to.

We grieve when someone we love dies, yes, but we also
grieve after divorce, a move away from a special city or
home, job transitions, separation from a loved one, serious
illness, and many other types of losses.

What causes grief is a threat to or severing of any attachment.

When we decide we want to have children, which can be from a very young age, we naturally begin to develop an attachment to our hopes and dreams for that child and the life we imagine we will share together. We look forward to the months of pregnancy and the birth. We think about what it will be like to have and love a baby and later a toddler and then a child and a teenager—and maybe beyond that, an adult child and eventually grandchildren.

That attachment includes grief when we discover that infertility stands in the way of all of those hopes and dreams.

Unlike most losses, however, infertility is often not an outward, tangible loss. Instead, it's the absence of something hoped for, perhaps even expected. It's an invisible loss. The heartbreak is hidden.

For those undergoing certain reproductive treatments, the loss may be more visible, but only in the isolated confines of the doctor's office. You may have seen follicles on the ultrasound screen, for example, or embryos in photographs.

Because your family members, friends, neighbors, and colleagues cannot see the loss, many probably don't recognize it. But as you know, the fact that the grief of infertility is not visible from the outside does not make it any less real or painful on the inside.

STIGMAS AND TABOOS

Compounding the invisibility of infertility loss are the stigmas associated with infertility. Our culture tends to judge fertility as normal and infertility as "abnormal." If we look to the past, we see the origins of this bias. Throughout human history, having children was typically associated with survival, wealth, and prestige. Larger families meant more children to work, earn money, and care for parents in old age.

At the same time, centuries-old religious beliefs promoting larger families also shaped our understanding of fertility.

Such bygone necessities of childbearing may be largely irrelevant today, but they still live on in our current (and often subconscious or unspoken) cultural and religious expectations about fertility.

Because of these longstanding traditions and values, and also because fertility is intertwined with taboos about sexuality, infertility was considered an unseemly subject until recently. Only in the last decade or so have we as a culture begun to discuss infertility more openly and see it for what it is—a very common physical challenge affecting both genders.

Still, both women and men physically affected by infertility may be made to feel "less than," even though the causes are not their fault and have nothing to do with their capacity or desire to be good, loving parents. Has this happened to you?

The stigmas can foster silence, which in turn can compound feelings of loneliness and isolation. Infertility is invisible, and the addition of silence to this invisibility typically creates even more pain and suffering.

CYCLICAL GRIEF AND THE TICKING CLOCK

In addition, infertility grief is also uniquely cyclical. While you are actively trying to have a baby, with or without reproductive assistance, each month is a new start. Will this be the month? Cautious hope gives way to disappointment and potentially despair every 28 days…and then the cycle starts all over again. The roller-coaster nature of this grief can make it even harder to withstand.

Finally, infertility grief can be made more complicated by the ticking biological clock. Some people don't decide to pursue having children until they are approaching the end of their fertility window, and if they aren't able to have a baby quickly, often find themselves feeling frustrated, confused, or ambivalent. What's more, in most types of grief, you can ease up on daily demands after a significant loss. You may be able to withdraw from nonessential commitments and lie low while you recuperate. But with infertility, there is often the need and the pressure to keep trying, month after month, especially if the remaining years of fertility are waning. You may have to plan every aspect of your life around your cycle. In addition to all your other life demands, how are you supposed to grieve and keep pursuing pregnancy at the same time? This high-pressure situation typically heightens anxiety, which we'll talk about soon.

Infertility grief is a uniquely difficult grief situation, but again, I want to remind you that you are not alone, and you are not powerless in your grief.

WHAT YOU MIGHT
THINK AND FEEL

"After a while, when you're not successful, you start to associate the word 'failure' every time you pee on a stick and it doesn't come out the right color. What starts out as a dream becomes a project that's all-consuming. Everywhere you look, women are pregnant. It becomes a very frustrating, frightening place."
— Brooke Shields

Infertility grief is typically made up of a wide variety of emotions. Remember that everything you think and feel about your struggles to have a baby is part of your grief. All of the thoughts and feelings are normal. And if you're having them, that means they're necessary for you, at least in the moment you're experiencing them.

After we review some of the most common thoughts and feelings, we'll talk about what you can *do* with those thoughts and feelings. That's where the empowering comes in.

SHOCK, DENIAL, AND NUMBNESS

Have you felt shocked or in denial about your infertility? It's understandable, because the cultural script says that having a baby is simple and natural (though the truth is that it's only simple sometimes, for some people).

You might also feel a sense of denial about your infertility grief. Have you found yourself wanting to push your grief aside and focus only on happy or "productive" things? Do you struggle with allowing yourself to feel sad when you feel sad, angry when you feel angry, etc.?

With infertility grief, it's also common for numbness to set in. Because of the monthly cyclical nature of fertility and infertility, things happen quickly. The pace can be fatiguing—and relentless. When our minds and hearts have to cope with so much every day, they begin to suppress strong feelings, good and bad, in an effort to simply survive. This is numbness—the dulling of everything.

CONFUSION AND DISORIENTATION

The grief of infertility can be so confusing. You may feel hopeful one moment and disappointed the next. You may not be sure what to hope for. You might feel confused about what caused the infertility. You might get caught up in all the doing and requirements of cycles and treatment and have no time to really get in touch with your thoughts and feelings.

And if you're not pursuing treatment, you may feel confused or at a loss about what to do next. In infertility grief, feeling disoriented and lost is common.

ANGER AND OTHER EXPLOSIVE EMOTIONS

If you've felt angry, rageful, blaming, resentful, or envious during your infertility journey, it's understandable, and it's OK. Like all feelings, these are normal.

With or without logical reasons, you might be mad at your partner or your family or friends. You might feel betrayed by your own body or your partner's body. You might be envious of people who've had children with ease or whose infertility treatments worked. You might blame God or doctors.

It might help you to know that explosive emotions are essentially feelings of protest. When something is happening that we don't want to be happening, we may express our objection with anger or blame. Essentially, we get mad instead of getting sad. Explosive emotions can feel better because they're more active than passive sadness or helplessness. But when we befriend our explosive emotions and dig deeper to really understand them, we generally uncover the sadness and fear they are protecting us from.

SHAME, GUILT, AND REGRET

Have you felt ashamed by your infertility? Have you felt inadequate, or like a failure? From my work with couples grieving infertility, I know that these feelings are really common and may dominate all other feelings at times. They are often and in large part due to the unfair social stigmas associated with infertility we discussed earlier.

Regret and guilt may also be part of the infertility grief experience. Regret may arise over past reproductive or sexual decisions. Guilt over things such as self-care choices, ambivalent feelings about childrearing, and competing demands for time and energy can also contribute. And any envious feelings of successful pregnancies of others may turn to shame at not being happy for them.

What's more, fertility decisions can also stir up these feelings. People pursuing treatment are often confronted with ethical choices such as reducing the number of embryos, or donating or disposing of unused embryos, for example. They may later feel uncertain or regretful about the decision they made, even though they were doing the best they could at the time.

Finally, the financial repercussions of fertility treatments may give rise to feelings of guilt and regret. Families often go deeply into debt for these expensive treatments. You might feel guilty about spending so much money as well as foreseeing the sacrifices your family may have to make well into the future to replenish your finances, or you might feel

The Grief of Infertility

guilty about worrying about money when it's being spent on such an important cause.

It's important for you to understand that while feelings are always valid, their causes may not always be. That is definitely true of feelings of inadequacy and shame. If they are part of your infertility grief experience, please know that you have the power to separate your clean pain from any stigma-created dirty pain (see page 40).

EMOTIONS, HORMONES, AND STRESS

For some but not all women, the emotions of infertility grief can sometimes be made more intense by reproductive-hormone fluctuations, especially among women who are receiving hormonal treatments. But studies have shown this correlation is relatively low.

For both women and men, the stress of infertility, on the other hand, is almost always part of the picture. Gender-neutral stress hormones such as adrenaline, cortisol, and norepinephrine heighten feelings of anger and fear. These hormones are more likely to be the culprits in any emotional intensification you may be experiencing than reproductive hormones.

Finding ways to manage stress that work for you is an essential part of your infertility grief self-care plan. We'll talk more about this on page 19.

ANXIETY, PANIC, AND FEAR

Infertility and anxiety typically go hand-in-hand. When you're following a rigorous and time-sensitive treatment regimen, when you're forced to pay attention to your body's every twinge, when you're worried about your ticking clock, when you live every day in uncertainty about the course your life will take…well, no wonder you're anxious.

Sex with your partner, which may have been an enjoyable stress reliever in the past, might now be contributing to your anxiety if it is regimented or associated with any feelings of failure or blame.

Anxiety and fear are closely related. Anxiety is a more generalized worry, while fear is a response to a specific threat. If you've miscarried before, you might be afraid of miscarrying again, for example. Your body produces the stress hormones adrenaline and cortisol (mentioned on the previous page) when you are afraid.

Fear and anxiety in infertility grief are normal, but they don't have to take over your life. They're hard on your body, your mind, your emotions, and your soul.

The Grief of Infertility

MANAGING STRESS IN INFERTILITY

Infertility is stressful. Treatment is stressful. Grief is stressful. All of this may be affecting you, your partner, and your relationship with each other.

Finding healthy, effective ways to manage your stress is incredibly important. Not only do stress hormones wreak havoc on your body, they also make life unpleasant at best.

One way to relax is through escapist activities like watching TV, reading, or surfing the internet. These work because they entertain and distract your stress-causing mind. Similarly, pursuits that occupy your body as well as your mind are also effective, but with the added benefits of physical movement. Examples of this include playing sports, making arts or crafts, cooking, and gardening.

It's healthy to distract your brain sometimes and move your body. But in addition to these tried-and-true stress management techniques, I hope you'll also learn to practice mindfulness. Mindfulness means training your awareness on the here and now, and regarding it with compassion, wonder, and hope. Mindfulness is about appreciating every minute of this precious life, and living it as slowly as you can. It's about cultivating an attitude of gratitude. And it's about making choices moment-to-moment about how to interact with the world in ways that don't just distract but rather feed your soul.

Practices such as meditation, yoga, tai chi, spending time in nature, reciting affirmations, keeping a gratitude journal, and many more can help you not only manage the stress of infertility but also live your best life. They're life-enhancing techniques no matter what your life issues are at any given moment.

SADNESS AND DEPRESSION

When you think of grief, you probably think of sadness. And indeed, your infertility grief may often make you heavyhearted, unhappy, discouraged, or just plain miserable.

Even though it's natural and understandable, sadness is often the hardest feeling to live with in infertility grief. It doesn't feel good, being sad. And because intense, active infertility grief can last for a span of many years, the sadness can be a heavy burden to carry for a long time.

People struggling with infertility grief are sometimes so caught up in their continued efforts to have a baby that they aren't fully aware of their sadness. They sometimes say they "don't feel like themselves anymore." If this applies to you, know that through attention to the six needs of mourning, which we'll start reviewing on page 23, you will learn to acknowledge your sadness as well as discover a path toward feeling like yourself again.

I always encourage grievers to see their primary-care providers if they think there is a chance they may be clinically depressed. Even if you are seeing fertility doctors all the time, your mental health may not be adequately supported. You should suspect your sadness has moved into clinical depression if you feel a sustained lack of self-worth or deep and unrelenting hopelessness. Therapy, medication, or a combination of both can help you out of this abyss. You deserve it.

HOPE AND HAPPINESS

Because the grief of infertility is often intermingled with the ongoing process of trying to have a baby or the pursuit of adoption, hope and happiness might be part of your day-to-day infertility story as well.

You might be trying a new treatment that promises good odds at success. Or maybe you're looking into surrogacy, fostering, or adoption. What's more, your life may also include a number of non-child-related experiences and activities you find satisfying or joyful.

Even when infertility grief is a significant part of your life, it is not *all* of your life. I hope that you are experiencing hope and happiness alongside your grief. It's healthy to actively seek out and cultivate moments of hope and happiness even amid the darkest times.

I would caution you, however, not to focus solely on hope. Some people struggling with infertility think that if they just keep pursuing the next treatment and try to stay positive at all times, everything will turn out OK. The trouble with this approach is that these people are denying their truth and their very normal and natural grief. They are jeopardizing their mental, physical, and spiritual health. You can and must befriend both your hope and your grief. It is a question of balance, and something you can work to achieve.

All of these feelings and more may be part of your infertility grief journey. Can you think of some that weren't covered? Next we'll talk about what you can *do* with your feelings to better integrate them into your life, now and into the future.

The Grief of Infertility

YOUR SIX NEEDS OF MOURNING

"Don't keep all your feelings sheltered—express them.
Don't ever let life shut you up."
— Dr. Steve Maraboli

We've talked about what grief is as well as many of the common feelings you might experience as part of your infertility grief. Now let's talk about mourning.

What's mourning? It's the outward expression of your inner thoughts and feelings of grief. Mourning is what you can choose to *do* with your grief. It's active engagement with your grief. And it's how you empower yourself to integrate your natural and necessary infertility grief into your ongoing life.

What I've learned from the thousands of grievers I've worked with over the years as well as my own life losses is that well-mourned grief becomes well-healed grief. And that is a worthy, life-affirming goal.

Following is a list of six tasks that I call the "needs of mourning." They're the things you'll do in the months to come to give awareness to your grief, express it, and move toward reconciling it. Keep in mind that even though they're numbered one through six, the needs of mourning are not really sequential steps (although it is important to focus on the first two initially). Instead, they're ongoing tasks that you'll be working on for many months and even years, sometimes singly, sometimes in twos or threes, and often all at once.

1. ACKNOWLEDGE THE REALITY AND APPROPRIATENESS OF YOUR GRIEF

You've probably experienced many of the thoughts and feelings we've covered so far in this book, but perhaps you never considered these thoughts and feelings "grief." Yet as I suggested, any attachment, when threatened or severed, gives rise to grief, and so you are indeed grieving.

Acknowledging your infertility grief is an essential first step. Your grief is real, and it is normal. It is appropriate, understandable, and legitimate.

So how do you meet this need of mourning? By giving yourself permission to grieve, and also by acknowledging the necessity of mourning. You accept your grief, and you accept the need to express your grief outside of yourself. Talking about the reality and appropriateness of your grief with someone who cares about you is a good way to work on this need.

The Grief of Infertility

Because, as we discussed, your loss is mostly invisible, it might help you to make it visible as you work on this need of mourning. For example, you could plant a tree, place a special houseplant, or hang a piece of art that represents your loss. This object can become a place to spend time whenever you are feeling the pain of your grief.

2. EMBRACE THE PAIN OF YOUR GRIEF

Grief is painful, but it's not "bad." It's a facet of your precious love and attachment, so how can it be bad? True, the circumstances causing the grief may be terrible, but the grief itself is normal and necessary.

We talked on page 9 about our culture's stigmas and taboos about infertility. Ironically, our culture has similar taboos about grief. We tend not to openly acknowledge loss. We encourage people to keep their feelings to themselves. We tell them to "keep their chin up," "get over it," and "look on the bright side." Two taboos together is double trouble.

But here's the thing: if you befriend your pain, it starts to soften. It may seem counterintuitive, but if you allow yourself to express your pain when you feel it welling up, you will ultimately feel better. This is because you are being honest with yourself, and honesty almost always feels "right." It's also because sharing your difficult thoughts and feelings outside of yourself is a relief. They've been building up pressure inside of you, and when they finally find a way out, there is a release of that pressure, at least for today.

So what are some ways you can mourn, or express, the pain of your infertility grief? You might cry. You might yell. You might talk to others, write in a journal, attend a support group, comment in an online forum, or make artwork. Whatever gives you that sense of release and comfort, do that—as often as you need to, for as long as you need to.

3. HONOR YOUR HOPES AND DREAMS

As we've emphasized, your grief is a result of the threat to or undoing of your hopes and dreams about having children and a certain kind of life. You have been attached to those hopes and dreams, perhaps for a long time. They were—and may continue to be—very special to you. They may have even felt like the most important wishes of your entire life.

Whether you are still pursuing this envisioned future or are now considering a different one, the hopes and dreams you cherished before infertility threw up a roadblock are still an essential part of your life story. And you honor them by exploring and expressing them.

Talking about jeopardized or dashed hopes and dreams with others who have experienced infertility is one way to meet this critical mourning need. Another is to share

The Grief of Infertility

openly with your partner about the future each of you had imagined. You might be surprised at and touched by the small, tender details each of you uniquely pictured. Seeing a compassionate counselor who can help you recount and fully understand those hopes and dreams is also an excellent option. Writing a long, heartfelt letter to your dreamed-of children will also help you explore and honor all of your hopes and dreams.

The more you explore and honor your long-held hopes and dreams about having children, the more likely it is you will gain momentum to work toward revised hopes and dreams that, even if they are different, share many of the same underlying feelings and goals.

4. REBUILD YOUR SELF-IDENTITY

Parenthood is a significant part of most people's self-identities. For many years, perhaps, you may have thought of yourself as a future mother or father in a particular kind of family situation. But now that that outcome seems delayed, less likely, changed, or not to be, you are forced to do the hard work of building a new way of thinking about your life to come, and possibly your future life with your partner as well.

If you are still uncertain about whether or not you will have a child, you can work on this need by asking yourself "what ifs" and then talking about the possible answers with a good listener who cares about you. What if I still don't have children (or another child) three years from now? What about five years? What about ten? What if I looked into adoption? What if I considered fostering? What if I explored bringing children into my life in other ways, such as through teaching, volunteering, or coaching?

If you have stopped pursuing pregnancy and childbirth, many but not all of the questions in the paragraph above also apply to your quest to rebuild your self-identity.

In addition, reconstructing your self-identity will involve taking stock of all the activities and relationships that give you a sense of meaning and purpose. How can you build your life around those things and less around things that don't matter as much to you? What have you always wanted to do but haven't yet? What are all the ways that you can add more depth, meaning, and joy into each and every day?

Rebuilding your self-identity is difficult work. It doesn't happen quickly or easily. But many infertility grievers I have counseled have taught me that active and ongoing work on this mourning need has helped them create full, satisfying lives and discover rewarding parts of themselves they never knew existed.

5. SEARCH FOR MEANING

All major loss experiences lead us to ponder the meaning of life and why things happen as they do. They also tend to make us examine our beliefs, questions, and doubts about the universe, God, religion, and spirituality.

During your infertility journey, if you've found yourself wondering why this had to happen to you, why others seemingly have so little trouble having children, or where God is in all of this, you're not alone. These are universal questions with no easy answers.

But this mourning need is not so much about finding the answers. It's about the search. It's essential to give yourself permission and time to search for meaning in your infertility experience. Taking even a few minutes each day to focus on spirituality is one excellent way to take positive action on this mourning need. Pray, meditate, attend services at a place of worship, read a spiritual text, have a philosophical conversation with a friend, walk a labyrinth, spend mindful time in nature—whatever centers you, calms you, and puts you in touch with your divine spark, do that.

Not only will regularly giving attention to this mourning need help you dissipate stress and feel better, it will also help you stay attuned to your inner compass, which always points to meaning and purpose.

6. RECEIVE ONGOING SUPPORT FROM OTHERS

To meet this final need of mourning, you'll need to muster the courage to break through the harmful taboos about both infertility and grief. You need and deserve the support of others as you live through and process this painful experience. To activate support, you'll need to open up about it. Tell select people how you are *really* feeling. Explain what's been happening. Unburden your heart.

It's OK to start small. Share your thoughts and feelings with just one person to begin with. Over time, you'll gradually find the courage and confidence to be open with more and more people.

Of course, you've probably already discovered by now that not everyone is equipped to be a good helper in grief. Most people have been shaped by our grief-avoiding culture, which prefers to deny or bottle up grief. But some people in your life—about one-third, in my experience—likely have the listening skills and empathy it takes to be present to you whenever you need to express what's in your mind and on your heart. Another third are typically neutral when it comes to grief support; they neither help nor hinder you, but might make good company for distracting or fun activities. And the final third can be toxic. These are the people who shame you, deplete your energy with their own dramas, or make you feel judged or dismissed. Avoid this last group as much as possible.

Remember that to be effective and sustainable, supportive relationships must be mutual. You need good listening ears and maybe a shoulder or two to cry on. Your empathetic listeners need the same thing—perhaps not today, but on some days. You can offer your support in return.

As I've mentioned, others who've had similar infertility experiences can serve as lifelines. Never underestimate the supportive, healing potential of shared pain. You may even develop deep, lifelong friendships with fellow infertility grievers you meet on your journey.

Working on the six needs of mourning is how you begin to better integrate your grief into your ongoing life. You don't stop grieving. Your grief isn't "cured" or "fixed." You don't "get over it." Instead, through active mourning you learn to make your infertility grief and your infertility story a part of who you are.

The amazing thing is that accommodating and befriending your pain eases it. It normalizes it, and eventually it allows your mind, heart, and soul to turn some of that grieving attention to other, hopeful things that spark and nurture meaning and purpose in your life.

ON ISOLATION AND SOLITUDE

Because of the invisibility of infertility and the taboos surrounding it, many people grieving infertility have shared with me they feel isolated and so lonely. Reaching out to others is the antidote. Be proactive about identifying your one-third of friends and family who are the true helpers (see page 30). Plug into support groups. Find a good counselor. Participate in community and social activities you enjoy.

Isolation is unhealthy, but occasional solitude will help you with mourning needs one through five. Solitude is intentional, mindful going within. It is shutting out the busyness and noise of the world temporarily so you can center yourself and hear the whispering of your soul.

Don't self-isolate, but do seek solitude now and then. How will you know the difference? The former feels lonely, while the latter feels restorative.

....

10 WAYS TO ACTIVELY MOURN YOUR INFERTILITY GRIEF TODAY

1. Text or email someone about how you're feeling—maybe someone who doesn't know yet. Make plans to meet for coffee so you can talk further in person.

2. Find an online infertility support forum and get connected. Review the Resources section at the end of this book.

3. Sit with your pain for 10 minutes. Set a timer if you want. Rest quietly, somewhere private and free of distractions. Feel your feelings about your infertility experience. Write down what you're thinking and feeling if you'd like to give that a try.

4. Schedule a date or a session with your partner to talk openly about each other's hopes and dreams related to family life and couple-hood or marriage.

5. Make a vision board that depicts your (changing?) hopes and dreams. Print out images you find online or tear them from magazines and glue them onto poster board.

6. Intentionally spend half an hour on something that gives you a sense of meaning and purpose.

7. What is something you've always wanted to do but never have? Take one small step today investigating it or making plans.

8. Take a spirit break. Do something you don't normally do that feeds your spirit and fills you with peace and wonder.

9. Meditate for 10 minutes. If you're unsure how, try a phone app like Calm or Breethe.

10. Consider what makes you feel most loved and supported— A heart-to-heart? Just hanging out together? Help with a household chore or a task? Words of encouragement?—and ask someone for that.

JILL'S STORY

The journey into infertility is long and unpaved. The first year is a waiting game of referrals and doctors reminding you to continue to try on our own. So the romance of the relationship takes a back seat while you're checking dates on calendars and scheduling in time with your spouse. Then come the grueling medical tests, filling in charts and health histories, and learning the best game plan to become a "family."

I cannot even remember how many early trips before the sun was up, 45 minutes into the city, to have blood drawn. I cannot remember how many days I showed up to work late because the line for blood work was long, filled with women just like me. I cannot count the amount of injections I placed into my belly or the bruises that took forever to disappear.

What I can remember is sitting by the phone every month, waiting for the nurse to call, already knowing that the results were negative, because I was already feeling crampy and moody—yet always hopeful that modern medicine had figured it out. I remember all the nights I cried myself to sleep, all the baby showers I went to with a smile on my face and a thoughtful gift under my arm. I remember wondering why some mothers had three or four children, and I remember praying for one of my own. So many prayers and promises to God to just make me a mom.

I avoided telling and sharing with anyone. I thought that I was protecting them from the hurt. I thought I was doing what was right. But I learned later that I had kept my struggle invisible from those who loved us. I was in hiding. The result of that hiding meant

I pushed all my emotions deep into the pit of my stomach. As I also learned that emotions cannot stay buried forever.

We are so blessed to have our son. We had a three-year journey to conceive him. And throughout the entire pregnancy, I worried about his health. It took so much time, money, and emotion to get to that stage. I worried every day he grew inside.

When he was two, we decided to start trying again. I honestly believed that modern science would know exactly what to do. After all, they mastered it the first time. I don't know what felt worse—trying to conceive the first time around, or failing permanently the second time. I felt like a complete failure.

When we decided to try to have our second, we set deadlines. We knew our limits financially. Having gone through it once before, we knew the emotional cost as well. So we were only going to spend so much, try for so long. We hit both of these limits. Devastated doesn't even begin to describe what it felt like. Crushed. All-consuming pain. Heartbreak. I had failed at giving a sibling to our son. The dreams of having lots of children were over.

We found out just before Thanksgiving. Ironic to find out around the holiday known for giving thanks. Yet we had this beautiful, healthy three-year-old. But I so desperately wanted another. We took the wishbone from the turkey. And we placed it under shallow soil in our backyard, where the sun would shine in the mornings. We planted a tulip maple tree. And we placed a Buddha statue of a baby at its base. I was able to look out at that special spot in the mornings as I sipped my coffee and watched the sun rise.

The journey started over a decade ago. And to be honest, it still aches. I still cry. But I no longer keep it private. I've begun to share our story. I share it when people question our decision to only have one child. I used to pause and shrug it off with a grin or a laugh. Now I'm honest. I share with people a piece of the reason why we are blessed to have one child. And we would have welcomed a carload if we could have. And although that one child can drive us nuts sometimes, I try never to take my motherhood moments for granted.

CARING FOR
YOUR WHOLE SELF

*"If you're struggling, you deserve to make self-care a priority.
Whether that means lying in bed all day, eating comfort food, crying,
sleeping, rescheduling plans, finding an escape through a good book,
watching your favorite TV show, or doing nothing at all—give
yourself permission to put your healing first. Feel your feelings,
breathe, and be gentle with yourself."*

— Daniell Koepke

If you've been busy with all the demands of everyday life plus fertility treatments/next steps plus your grief, your plate is probably already spilling over. The purpose of this section is not to put more on your plate but instead to make it more manageable—and, I hope, more meaning-centric at the same time.

Perhaps you've realized already that grief is not just an emotional journey. It's also a physical, cognitive, social, and spiritual experience. And so, when you care for yourself in grief, it's essential to care for yourself in all of these ways.

Your life is better when you balance all of your needs and care for yourself holistically.

CARING FOR YOUR PHYSICAL SELF

If you are a woman who has been trying to have a baby, especially if you have been through fertility treatments, you may feel fatigued, sore, tense, and run-down. You may also have an ambivalent relationship with your body right now.

Whether or not you are the one who has been trying to have the baby, your grief also naturally impacts your body. Grief tends to make people tired and even achy. You might be catching germs more easily, since your immune system may have been weakened by all the stress. You might be having gastrointestinal issues, sleep problems, higher blood pressure, and other bodily grief symptoms.

Your body is telling you it needs TLC, and now is the time to listen. If you're feeling overwhelmed, ask others to help you with physical care. Getting enough quality sleep is the highest priority. If you're not sleeping well or enough, take measures to enhance your sleep. See a physician or work on any barriers. Eating healthy food and drinking enough water will also help establish a baseline of physical health. Talk to your partner about ways to support both of you with good nutrition. Gentle but regular exercise is important as well.

Even a ten-minute walk twice a day can make a remarkable difference.

Once the basics are in place, consider other physical self-care rituals that might improve your quality of life. Naps, massages, manicures, acupuncture, and new physical activities—kite-flying? paddle-boarding? dancing?—can all help you achieve a healthy balance between the demands of infertility and grief on the one hand and enjoyment of life on the other.

CARING FOR YOUR COGNITIVE SELF

Grief as well as the infertility diagnosis and treatment gauntlet can leave you feeling muddled and unable to think clearly. If you've been having trouble completing even simple tasks or remembering new information, for example, this is normal.

As much as possible, your brain probably needs some rest right now. This is one area where you may be able to offload some of the tasks and responsibilities overfilling your plate. Consider dropping any optional projects and obligations for the time being. Say no to invitations that feel overwhelming. Simplify, simplify, simplify. The more you're able to simplify your life right now, the more you may also free up time for extra physical, emotional, social, and spiritual self-care.

Tasks and activities that fully immerse you in that feeling of "flow," on the other hand, are good for your brain. These are things that make you feel engaged and alive. If you're not sure if an undertaking is a good idea or a bad one, ask yourself if it will deplete you or help restore you.

CARING FOR YOUR EMOTIONAL SELF

In the "Your Six Needs of Mourning" section, starting on page 23, I suggested a number of ways to express your thoughts and feelings of infertility grief. Always remember that sharing your feelings is the foundation of good emotional self-care, especially when it comes to grief.

If your emotions are particularly tender, or easily brought to the surface, that simply means they need your time and attention right now. Be sure to give them some dedicated awareness each day. Try sitting or walking in solitude while you pay attention to whatever you're feeling. Ask yourself what in particular the feeling is associated with and why. Name the feeling.

As you're attending to your emotions, it may help you to distinguish between *"clean pain"* and *"dirty pain."* What's the difference? Clean pain is the normal pain that follows difficult life experiences such as infertility. Dirty pain is the damaging, multiplied pain we create when we catastrophize, judge ourselves, or allow ourselves to be judged by others.

In infertility grief, the threat to or loss of hopes and dreams creates clean pain. But the stigmas surrounding infertility can cause dirty pain as well. If you feel you did something wrong, for example, or that something is wrong with you, dirty pain is being heaped on top of the clean pain. You can learn to unburden yourself of the dirty pain. Dirty pain isn't fair, and it isn't based on the truth. Discussing dirty pain with someone who understands can help you be kinder to yourself as well as more effective in your life journey.

TRIGGERS AND GRIEFBURSTS

In grief, triggers are cues that make you think about and feel your loss. Depending on where you are in your infertility journey and the specifics of your unique hopes and dreams, your grief might be triggered by a certain song, the sight of a pregnant woman or a baby, a TV commercial depicting a sappy family moment, a social media post, or just about anything!

When you encounter a trigger, you might feel a sudden, unexpected wave of intense grief. I call these normal rushes of pain "griefbursts." Sometimes you might be surprised at the severity of the pain. Griefbursts usually need your attention for just a few minutes. It might help you to make a plan for what you'll do the next time you experience one. Many grievers like to retreat to somewhere private and have a good cry. Others feel comforted by reaching out to a special listener.

Just as joy will sometimes burst in on you without warning, so will grief. Both are facets of love, and both must be received with grace.

....

CARING FOR YOUR SOCIAL SELF

Humans are social creatures. Whether you consider yourself an extrovert or an introvert, you need people and relationships in your life. After all, it is our relationships that give our lives the most meaning.

But social connections often suffer during the infertility journey. If you're overly busy, you may have had little extra time to spend with family and friends. If your energy has been low or your emotions draining, you may have felt like cocooning yourself at home. The difficulties of answering questions about when you're going to have a baby or spending time with others who have young children may have caused you to avoid family or social gatherings.

It may be necessary and healthy to spend some time in solitude right now (see page 32), and it's OK to take a break from attending baby showers and other gatherings, yet your social self also craves love and support. Remember the sixth need of mourning—receive ongoing support from others? Your grieving self needs other people. You need kindness, affirmation, and empathy right now. To get those things, you'll need to reach out to other people, and accept their

The Grief of Infertility

support when they reach out to you.

Try to build at least one meaningful social interaction into each day. Not counting the people who live in your household, actively seek to share a conversation, a meal, or an activity with someone you care about and who cares about you. It might just be a brief touching-base texting conversation, it might be a get-your-mind-off-your-problems game of golf, or it might be a heart-to-heart discussion. As long as you're revealing at least a little bit about what's going on inside you during the interaction, it counts.

CARING FOR YOUR SPIRITUAL SELF

Grief is many things, but I believe it's most of all a spiritual journey. It forces us to consider what we value most in life, and it encourages us to ask profound questions about the meaning of life and why we're here. The deepest grief comes from threats to or the loss of people and attachments that we attribute the most meaning to. And "meaning" is a spiritual concept.

And yet I've observed that people tend to make caring for their spiritual selves a low priority. It often seems optional somehow. Is that true of you? If so, I'm asking you to flip that thinking around. Caring for your spiritual self should be your highest priority right now. If you're caring well for your spirit, caring for the other aspects of yourself—physical, cognitive, emotional, and social—will naturally fall into place.

How you care for your spirit is up to you. The suggestions I offered in the "search for meaning" section on page 29 are all good ways to care for your spiritual self. You may need to try a number of things to find a combination that works for you. Again, whatever centers you, calms you, and puts you in touch with your divine spark, do that.

I urge you to dedicate at least 15 minutes each and every day to caring for your spirit. The more you care for your spiritual self in the months and years to come, the more likely you are to find pursuits and nurture relationships that fill your life with deeply rewarding meaning and purpose.

INTEGRATING GRIEF AND HOPE INTO YOUR ONGOING LIFE

"The trick is to enjoy life. Don't wish away your days, waiting for better ones ahead."

— Marjorie Pay Hinckley

One of the great secrets of life is that we can choose to bring awareness to difficulties and to joys at the same time. Life is rarely all "good" or all "bad." Instead, it is a jumbled, ever-changing mixture of everything all at once. And to live authentically means to be present and open to all of it.

Although grief may understandably drag us under on particularly painful days, most of the time we can embrace both our grief and our happiness—and be mindful of all the seemingly mundane (but in fact remarkable!) things in between.

Plus, learning to befriend our grief as a normal and necessary part of our love can be so freeing. We're free to be vulnerable. We're free to live life deeply. We're free to take chances and to always be reaching out for meaning, purpose, and love.

As you learn to befriend your grief—and it is indeed a learning process that takes time and conscious, repeated focus—it is also essential to simultaneously befriend hope. Think of grief and hope as a seesaw, and you're allowing the seesaw to go up and down with the natural weight of whatever's happening on any given day...but you're also working to maintain some degree of leveling of the seesaw over the course of the weeks and months.

Hope is forward-looking. It is an expectation of a good that is yet to be. We've talked about the fact that your infertility grief has arisen from your hopes about having and raising children. Unfortunately, infertility is standing between your present and your expectations of that future.

Yet you also have other hopes for your future. Perhaps your child-related hopes for your future are changing or evolving. Maybe you're coming to think about the concept of family itself in different ways. You may also have great hopes about your career, volunteer efforts, travel, and life celebrations, just to name a few.

If you believe that your future will include moments of joy, love, and meaning, you already have within you that spark of hope. You can grow that spark into a flame by intentionally building hope into each day.

How do you build hope? Here are a few ways:

- By taking part in activities you care about

- By engaging in spiritual practices

- By making future plans that excite you and that you know you will enjoy

- By helping others

- By interacting with families of all different kinds and bearing witness to their love

- By taking care of your body, your mind, your heart, your social connections, and your soul

The hopes and dreams you have had for children and a certain kind of family life are precious and will always live inside you. The changing hopes and dreams you are now nurturing are no less precious. In fact, you might say that hopes and dreams built on the present moment are always exceptionally beautiful and meaningful because they are the most alive with momentum and possibility.

Your infertility grief is part of you. If you nurture it, your hope is also part of you. And the beauties and challenges of whatever this day brings are part of you. All of it belongs.

A FINAL WORD

"Here is the world. Beautiful and terrible things
will happen. Do not be afraid."
— Frederick Buechner

It's true that fear is a natural and normal part of grief. If
you have been fearful or anxious as part of your infertility
journey, I don't want you to be ashamed of your fear. But I
do want to emphasize that befriending your grief tames it.
Over time, it makes it less painful and less fearful.

You do not need to be afraid of grief. It is simply your love in
a different form. As you live the remainder of your precious
days, more beautiful and terrible things will happen, as they
do to all of us. Actively mourning the inevitable pain as it
arises will help you stay present to and fully engaged in your
one, singular life, no matter what happens.

I wish you a mindful appreciation of life. I wish you many
wonderful experiences to come. I wish you grace and hope
and joy and meaning. And I wish you love, which is the
deepest meaning we mortals are privileged to experience.

I realize that in wishing you love and attachment, I'm also wishing you grief, since the two are conjoined. And yet, of course, still I wish you love. The people I've counseled who've journeyed through infertility grief also wish you love. Godspeed.

THE INFERTILITY GRIEF
BILL OF RIGHTS

TEN SELF-COMPASSIONATE PRINCIPLES

Though you should reach out to others as you journey through your grief, you should not feel obligated to accept the unhelpful responses you may receive from some people. You are the one who is grieving, and as such, you have certain "rights" no one should try to take away from you.

The following list is intended both to empower you to befriend your grief and to decide how others can and cannot help.

1. *You have the right to experience your own unique grief.*
   No one else will grieve infertility exactly the same way you do. So, when you turn to others for help, don't allow them to tell you what you should or should not be feeling.

2. *You have the right to talk about your grief.*
   Talking about your grief will help you heal. Seek out others who will allow you to talk as much as you want,

as often as you want, about your grief. If occasionally you don't feel like talking, you also have the right to be silent, as long as you're not isolating yourself.

3. *You have the right to feel many different emotions.*
Confusion, numbness, fear, guilt, and anger are just a few of the emotions you might feel as part of your infertility grief journey. Others may try to tell you that feeling angry, for example, is wrong. Don't take these judgmental responses to heart. Instead, find listeners who will accept your feelings without condition.

4. *You have the right to be tolerant of your physical and emotional limits.*
In addition to your regular demands and possibly infertility treatments, your feelings of loss and sadness will probably leave you feeling fatigued. Respect what your body and mind are telling you. Get daily rest. Eat balanced meals. Take care of yourself with compassion and tenderness.

5. *You have the right to experience "griefbursts."*
Sometimes, out of nowhere, a powerful surge of grief may overcome you. This can be frightening, but it is normal and natural. Find someone who understands and will let you talk it out.

6. *You have the right to break through stigmas.*
   The stigmas surrounding infertility and grief might make
   it harder for you to talk openly about your experiences.
   Talk and express your feelings openly anyway. It will help
   you, and it will also help our culture.

7. *You have the right to embrace your spirituality.*
   Explore and express your spirituality in ways that feel
   right to you. Allow yourself to be around people who
   understand and support your beliefs and values. If you
   feel angry at God, find someone to talk with who won't be
   critical of your feelings of hurt and abandonment.

8. *You have the right to search for meaning.*
   You may find yourself asking, "Why did this have to
   happen? Why me?" Some of your questions may have
   answers, but some may not. And watch out for the
   clichéd responses some people may give you. Comments
   like, "It's God's will," "There are so many children in need
   of a good home," At least you didn't lose a child," or
   "Think of all the things you still have to be thankful for"
   are not helpful, and you do not have to accept them.

9. *You have the right to honor your hopes and dreams.*
   You are grieving a threat or end to cherished hopes and
   dreams. You have the right to honor those hopes and
   dreams by sharing them with others, writing them

down, and discussing them with your partner. You also have the right to create new hopes and dreams if and when you are ready.

10. *You have the right to live a life of meaning and joy.*
    You have encountered a very difficult roadblock in your life. This roadblock has caused you deep grief, which you must mourn thoroughly. But even as you are grieving and mourning, you also have the right to move forward in life with meaning and joy.

RESOURCES

Adoption Network, adoptionnetwork.com

American Society for Reproductive Medicine, reproductivefacts.org

Choice Moms, choicemoms.org

Creating a Family, creatingafamily.org

International Council on Infertility Information Dissemination, inciid.org

RESOLVE: The National Infertility Association, resolve.org

The Seleni Institute, seleni.org

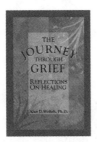

The Journey Through Grief
REFLECTIONS ON HEALING | SECOND EDITION

This revised, second edition of *The Journey Through Grief* takes Dr. Wolfelt's popular book of reflections and adds space for guided journaling, asking readers thoughtful questions about their unique mourning needs and providing room to write responses.

ISBN 978-1-879651-11-1 • 152 pages • hardcover • $21.95

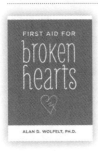

First Aid for Broken Hearts

Life is both wonderful and devastating. It graces us with joy, and it breaks our hearts. If your heart is broken, this book is for you. Whether you're struggling with a death, break-up, illness, unwanted life change, or loss of any kind, this book will help you both understand your predicament and figure out what to do about it.

ISBN: 978-1-61722-281-8 • softcover • $9.95

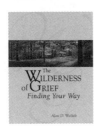

The Wilderness of Grief
A BEAUTIFUL, HARDCOVER GIFT BOOK VERSION OF
UNDERSTANDING YOUR GRIEF

The Wilderness of Grief is an excerpted version of *Understanding Your Grief*, making it approachable and appropriate for all mourners. This concise book makes an excellent gift for anyone in mourning. On the book's inside front cover is room for writing an inscription to your grieving friend.

ISBN 978-1-879651-52-4 • 112 pages • hardcover • $15.95

All Dr. Wolfelt's publications can be ordered by mail from:
Companion Press, 3735 Broken Bow Road, Fort Collins, CO 80526
(970) 226-6050 • www.centerforloss.com

NOTES:

NOTES:

ABOUT THE AUTHOR

Alan D. Wolfelt, Ph.D., is a respected author and educator on the topics of companioning others and healing in grief. He serves as Director of the Center for Loss and Life Transition and is on the faculty at the University of Colorado Medical

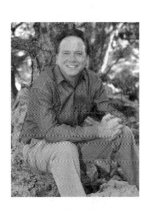

School's Department of Family Medicine. Dr. Wolfelt has written many bestselling books on healing in grief, including *Understanding Your Grief, Healing Your Grieving Heart*, and *The Mourner's Book of Hope*. Visit www.centerforloss.com to learn more about grief and loss and to order Dr. Wolfelt's books.